NO MORE CASUALTIES

BREAKING THE GLASS CEILING IN THE CARE PROFESSION

Barry
Be inspired to live you dream!
Shirley
28/03/12

SHIRLEY BAAH-MENSAH

FastPrint Publishing
www.fast-print.net/store.php

No More Casualties
Breaking Through The Glass Ceiling
In The Care Profession

ISBN 978-178035-015-8

Edited By
Roy Stannard

Cover design and layout
David Springer
Designs4me.com

First published 2011 by
FASTPRINT PUBLISHING
Peterborough, England.

Dedication

I would like to dedicate this book to all BME nurses, midwives, health visitors, social workers and teachers for their commitment to finding fulfilment and success at the work place.

Acknowledgements

I give special thanks to my husband and children for their support and belief in me and for their priceless backing in all I have achieved over the years.

I appreciate all the coaches and mentors in my life who have supported and encouraged me in making my vision a reality.

Also I acknowledge all my friends and colleagues for their continuous support in all my endeavours.

A big thank you to the editor and all who have worked to see this project completed

Contents

CONTENT **PAGES**

Foreword

It can be extremely disheartening when a person with ability and commitment experiences constant obstacles that prevent them from reaching their desired career goal. It is clear that there are many examples of barriers that can block advancement within any organisation, including the National Health Service. There is evidence that ethnicity is one such factor and why this book could be of great assistance to Black and Minority Ethnic staff working within the NHS. Shirley is to be congratulated for pulling together strategies that individuals can use to advance their career.

Those of us who have managed to reach senior positions appreciate the support and advice we have received from individuals who have identified our talents and possible contributions that we can offer to the organisation. When asked to reflect back upon my own career and offer tips on 'how to succeed' the following suggestions come to mind.

Identify what you feel really strongly about, are prepared to work hard at and even maybe receive recognition as an expert. For me this centred on improving services for families affected by sickle cell disorder and currently, campaigning for a statue of Mary Seacole.

Whilst being clear about your strengths you will also need to have a thick enough skin to take on board your weaknesses. This can be assisted by listening to what others may have to say in this matter! It may hurt but it can be of great assistance in your future development.

Ensuring you have personal and professional support networks is vital to avoid negative emotional experiences taking hold and slowly building up to become a destructive personal force. These networks may be formal and informal and consist of both likeminded individuals and those who come from a very different cultural and professional background. Identify individuals who you admire because of their achievements and ask them to become your mentor, they can only say no! Be prepared to listen to what they say, however tough. In addition real mentors, friends and colleagues are those who point out to you signs of change in your behaviour that may be due to depression or bottled up anger. They are also the ones who are the first to genuinely congratulate you on your successes.

Taking care of your personal wellbeing is equally important as striving to advance your career. We are more prone to conditions such as high blood pressure and diabetes so therefore need to set aside time to review our nutrition, get up off that sofa and exercise as well as making time to relax with family and friends.

Finally take heart from the words of Jamaican born Mary Seacole in London in 1854. Following the last of five rejections of her offer to nurse soldiers in the Crimean war she recalled that: 'A good night's rest had served to strengthen my determination. Let what might happen, to the Crimea I would go.' The rest, as they say, was history!

[www.maryseacoleappeal.org.uk]

PROFESSOR ELIZABETH N ANIONWU

CBE FRCN, EMERITUS PROFESSOR OF NURSING,

THAMES VALLEY UNIVERSITY AND VICE-CHAIRPERSON;

MARY SEACOLE MEMORIAL STATUE APPEAL

Introduction

'You cannot build character and courage by taking away a man's initiative and independence'.

Abraham Lincolm.

Your decision to explore this book probably means that you feel that too many Black and Minority Ethnic (BME) career casualties have happened already. It's likely that you want to know how to avoid more in the future. So how?

This book will help you discover how to break through the glass ceiling, using its techniques to fast track to the successful future you want. *No More Casualties* unpicks how health and social care organisations work. Knowing this will re-enfranchise you. You will take control of your career development and set about progressing to your full potential.

The personal experience of people in the National Health Service (NHS) over many years, and research centred on equality and diversity issues within it, suggest that, although trying hard to be seen as an equal opportunities employer, the NHS fails to deliver this ethos throughout the organisation. As a result, some people are more successful than others, and Black and Minority Ethnic nurses and doctors in particular struggle to travel the road to success. It is indisputable that a disproportionate number of BME in the care profession have become casualties in the NHS, usually having to work 40 years or more beneath the glass ceiling to receive equitable rewards - and to qualify for a living pension when they retire.

There are good reasons why BME employees in health and social care are not found in the Organisation's boardrooms. This book focuses on how the BME workforce is directly impacted on by the operational policies of the NHS, and explores how they can influence change in these policies, and in the process narrow the gulf between themselves and their white counterparts. The methods discussed here are designed for staff in health and social care, as well as others from different walks of life who want to manage their own career development and perform to their full potential.

No one disputes that the BME are intelligent people with sound clinical skills, knowledge and experience, who, given equality of access, will perform well at senior managerial level. This book sets out to explain how political expediency, organisational culture and the behaviour of decision makers all conspire to fetter creativity and initiative, and turn BMEs into career casualties. *No More Casualties* makes clear to politicians and decision-makers that discrimination does impede many BME staff. It also endeavours to show those at the receiving end of discrimination that the process of changing the status quo starts with them.

Many good men and women have fought tirelessly to eradicate discrimination and racism in the NHS. The time has come for BME people to take the responsibility of making it happen for themselves – by adopting a bottom up approach to change.

The power to do this is already in place. This book's aim is to equip the individuals who need them with the skills to harness that power.

The first section deals with some of the major reasons why large numbers of the BME workforce are career casualties and have been so for institutional reasons for a long time. The second suggests solutions ending with a call to arms to break through the glass ceiling to the rarefied climes of the management chamber above.

Even those with a rudimentary interest in the NHS will be aware that it was created in 1948, over 60 years ago. It is the third largest employer in the world with 1.3 million employees, (comparable to the Russian Army), working collectively to improve the health of the Nation. This monolithic structure has stumbled at times under the sheer weight of this challenge. Most people would agree that, as the organisation has evolved, the challenges it faces have grown with it, especially in the area of funding to quality ratios - and in its value for money offering.

All recent studies agree that discrimination in the NHS is economically counter-productive. Where it is found, output falls whilst migration outwards occurs in the groups discriminated against. Another outcome is that health needs of local people, especially people from the same ethnic groups as disenchanted, departing nurses stop being met. Economists are aware of this and have advised the NHS not to merely pay lip service to equal opportunities among the workforce, but to deliver inclusive opportunities for

BME workers. The NHS, through its senior managers, needs to demonstrate that diversity and equal opportunity is embraced throughout the workforce, amongst patients and within all its services.

NHS employees are its most valuable assets and, as such, should be prized. Working within the care industry is a highly pressurised experience. Dealing with critically ill people, frequent emergencies, life threatening conditions and complex social needs, expose workers to high levels of stress. In consequence, it is imperative that the NHS, through its managers, behaves in a way that visibly works to reduce these stress levels rather than add to them. Inequality in any setting is bad; inequalities in health care are inherently damaging to the Nation. The question is: How do we begin to calculate the cost of inequality in terms of lost opportunities, hidden discrimination, open bullying and harassment among the workforce?

In this book, we will explore ways of climbing the career ladder by re-calibrating some of these inequalities. The book will also assist the reader to design their own chosen futures and pursue goals that will serve as signposts along the way. This information will provide a fresh perspective on career development, increase levels of satisfaction, and enhance participation in the Health Service - and other areas of employment.

Section One

Care Profession Casualties - The Game Untold

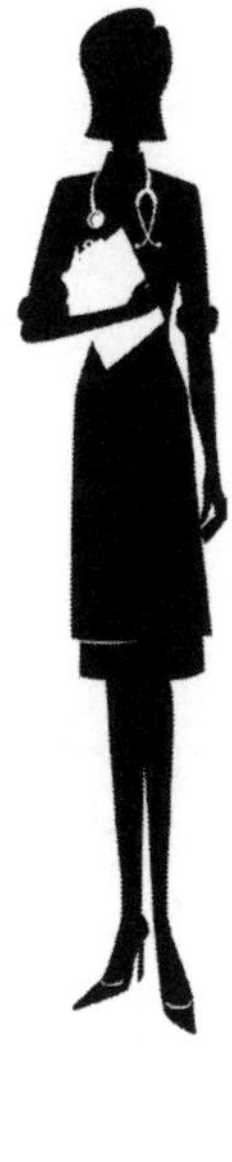

CHAPTER 1

Politics, Politics, Politics

'Concerns for man and his welfare must always form the chief interest of all technical endeavours. Never forget this in the midst of your diagrams and equations.'

Albert Einstein

THE POLITICAL GAME

Day Three after the 2010 General Election. The nurses on Seacole Ward, a medical unit in Nightingale Hospital, looked subdued, their heads bent in deep political discussion. The Sister in charge, Sister Callaghan, emerged from her office twice that morning to ask nurses to concentrate, look after patients and stop discussing politics. On the same day, a West African nurse, Adenike Oladejide (re-christened Jane by her English colleagues) started an Adaptation Course on Seacole Ward. West Indian Nurse, Sarah James was asked to work with Jane as her mentor. She was to teach and supervise her for the six months of her Adaptation Course that would licence her to practise as a nurse in the UK. Jane, new to the NHS and new on the ward, was amazed at how the political mood of the country was impacting on the nurses on duty.

'Why are they so worried about who the next Prime Minister will be?' she asked. 'What have nurses got to do with politicians?'

Sarah sympathised with Jane for not realising the extent to which politics and the health service were entwined - both in service delivery and in the politics of the workplace. She took the opportunity to explain to her student how the NHS continues to be a political 'hot potato' and that, just as there was a national general election every four years, so there was usually a major overhaul of the Health Service. It had become common practice for politicians to make major policy changes in the public sector every few years - in local authorities, the police, education, health and social care.

'In my opinion,' Sarah continued, 'the NHS is vulnerable to cuts and reforms because it currently costs £104 billion to run and that figure is set to rise. So the political impetus for politicians to demand economies in services is high.'

Since Jane was at the start of her career as a nurse in the NHS, Sarah thought it wise to give her a short history lesson on the founding origins of the organisation. She started by explaining the three main aims of the NHS to her student:

> ***to meet the health needs of everyone;***
> ***to provide care free at the point of delivery;***
> ***to provide care based on clinical need, not ability to pay.***

Achieving these three main pillars of the original Aneurin Bevan vision for the NHS was an almost impossible challenge and provided a constant thorn in the flesh of politicians. Universal access to health care in the NHS has always been popular with the public, but funding the phenomenal cost of delivering that model of care has been difficult. Attempts to alter the structure of the organisation and the way care is delivered, (which economists have argued was flawed from the outset), proved taxing, literally. Sarah explained that, because the NHS is tax-funded, it is a sacred cow and therefore a sensitive area for change. Politicians are dissuaded from initiating major reform as any attempt to implement changes unpopular with the public would see them voted out of office.

'Almost everybody at some point in their lives will need medical attention,' Sarah went on, 'so everyone has a vested interest in what happens to the NHS. If the public think the Government has got it wrong, they have the power to change that Government at election time. The public really do have power, and nurses could harness this power if they understood which levers to pull. The public usually supports nurses.'

Soon it was break time, and as Sarah and Jane went into the staff room to grab a hurried drink, Mary, the second nurse on the ward, joined them for coffee. The three nurses continued with their conversation on the political state of the NHS. Mary, who enjoyed a good debate, enthusiastically joined in the conversation. She thought politicians sometimes tried too hard to achieve the complex blend of high quality service and cost effective care. She disliked the fact that the NHS was plagued with reports and new initiatives, and many of these initiatives were introduced prematurely before being fully thought through and road-tested. Mary was concerned that there was a revolving door of policies, especially after a general election, and that this was confusing for staff. The public sector workforce was made to work through a plethora of bottlenecked red tape, with 'all change' being shouted every five minutes.

'Every worker in the NHS knows the saying,' laughed Mary, 'that the only thing that's constant is change!'

New to all this, Jane wondered why so many of these changes were necessary. The more worldly wise Sarah observed that sometimes changes were made because there was a 'new king', and new laws followed. Health experts opposed the political changes, but no one listened. The new plans were always implemented.

'The most common accusation levelled against politicians for making some of these unnecessary changes,' Mary explained, 'is that they're money-driven rather than care-driven.'

Jane listened carefully as Sarah expanded upon the plight of NHS workers caught up in a major recession. To provide a taste of the volume of documents, initiatives, directives and policies that nurses had to contend with, Sarah took her to a little room attached to the staff room where a document library was kept for the workforce. Jane was staggered by the sheer volume of policies that nurses had been expected to implement in the past decade alone. She asked for copies of some of them to read at home as part of her commitment to know more about how the system operated in Britain.

'Take a deep breath', Sarah said. 'There have been over 500 health policy documents issued in the past decade.' A few of the major ones include:

- ***2000 The NHS Plan***
- ***2002 Health Visitor and School Nurse Development Resource Packs***
- ***2003 Liberating The Talents***
- ***2003 Tackling Inequalities In Health***
- ***2004 Every Child Matters***
- ***2004 The Children's Act***
- ***2004 Choosing Health – making healthier choices easier***
- ***2004 NHS Improvement Plan***
- ***2005 The Common Assessment Framework***
- ***2005 The NHS Forward Plan***
- ***2005 Choosing Health: White Paper***
- ***2005 Tackling Health Inequalities: a status report on the programme for action***
- ***2007 Mental Health Act***
- ***2008 Our Health, Our Care, Our Say: a new direction for community services***
- ***2009 Healthy Child Programme***

> ***2010 Equity And Excellence Liberating The NHS***

Sarah sighed, 'The real difficulty with these repeated shifts in NHS policy direction is the stress they create in staff. The "go" button is often pressed too quickly before the real ramifications of that decision are considered - bureaucrats fiddle, Rome burns. Nurses may be delivering care in accordance with the old system while waiting for the new one to start. The patient on the other hand arrives expecting something new, and complains because they're not receiving the care package promised by the politicians!'

As the nurses walked back to the ward after their coffee break, Mary said that the changes often meant cut backs in staffing, and this caused high levels of anxiety among employees as everyone wondered 'who's next?'

Day Five after the General Election. The mood on Seacole was still sober. The morning shift had started and nurses were doing their rounds in the bays, seeing patients. Sarah and her student, Jane, were working together, but instead of talking shop, they were discussing who the next Prime Minster would be.

'Where I come from, this wouldn't be happening,' Jane smiled. 'In my country, unless the ruling party wishes to leave, no one can force them out. The ruling party wins every election unless there's a "coup d'état". So all these negotiations around forming a coalition government would never happen there.'

'Things are done differently in England,' Sarah replied. 'The current situation is unique. The deal done in smoke-filled rooms will lead to policy-making and, all being well, the politicians will come up with a workable solution soon. Let's hope it's the right one for all our sakes. We're living in a very special era.'

'What do you mean?' Jane asked.

'This year,' Sarah said, 'is the end of the first decade of the third millennium. It's been full of surprises, extraordinary events and extreme phenomena - natural and man-made. This is the decade when Barack Obama became the first black President of the US. Let's hope the outcome of our election in the UK is equally as history-making!'

Sister Callaghan came out of the office for the first time that morning and demanded across the bay, 'Are you two working or chatting?' She had a list of tasks for the two nurses and kept looking at her watch impatiently. By the end of their shift, the pair were only too glad to hand over to their colleagues on the late shift, go home and watch the news for an update on the political situation.

The next day, Sarah and Jane were working the afternoon shift and had heard the news that Britain had elected a coalition government: the Conservatives and Liberal Democrats had forged an agreement for the sake of the Country – Con Lib, as it was being called. This outcome was something that more than half the electorate had not experienced before. The portents were not good. Past experience suggested that governments of all the talents had not been very effective.

Sarah, who had recently bought a flat, was particularly anxious. Folding in a bedsheet corner, she observed, 'The global recession has caused a credit crunch that's affecting most households and businesses. I'm not happy with these chalk and cheese political alliances forming to govern us. This really is a new political era. Two parties for the price of one in government! All we can do now is watch this space and hope for the best.'

As the ward wasn't very busy, Sarah and Jane decided to have an early tea break before the evening routine started. Jane had more questions about the link between the NHS and politics. Sarah told her that Britain had seen drastic changes over the 60-year life span of the NHS. As demographic and societal faultlines shifted in the country, consumer preferences evolved, yet demand for quality was constant. New technology and competition in the market place were driving change in every area of life, including work.

Sarah remembered when she first became a nurse. 'We used to say, "become a nurse and you'll have a job for life." That isn't true any more. There is no job security in any profession - including nursing.'

THE CASUALTIES

Now a month into her adaptation course, Jane was enjoying herself. She was eager, a fast learner and observant. But as she went around the different departments building her experience, she became aware of a problem that had plagued the NHS since its inception.

'Where is the diversity in leadership and senior management in the NHS - and the teaching university?' she asked, puzzled.

Sarah feigned that she hadn't heard Jane's question. They continued working, but when their eyes met, Jane asked again why there were no BME in senior management in the hospital. Sarah knew she couldn't avoid the issue.

'There's no short answer to that,' she began. 'It would probably take a whole year for me to give you a proper understanding of race and equality issues in the NHS.'

Then she remembered that they had booked onto a course the next day. 'I think it would be better for us to talk about this tomorrow when we're training.'

'Why?' Jane frowned. 'Are you saying we shouldn't talk about racism on the ward?'

Sarah sighed. 'Racism in the NHS is the elephant in the room - everyone knows it's there but nobody wants to mention it.'

Wednesday morning arrived. Sarah and Jane attended the training day at the local school of nursing. It's purpose? To explore how professionals can involve patients in the planning and provision of care - via a patient/public partnership to achieve service delivery. Although London was now multicultural and the service provision of the NHS attempted to reflect this, it was difficult to engage people from non-white backgrounds in discussions about their care. Committees and steering groups in the Health Service were predominantly Caucasians not BME. Budget holders of equality and diversity departments in the organisation were usually Caucasian too, with a limited understanding of the cultural needs of the people they were serving.

Jane wanted to know why nurses from BME groups weren't enthusiastic about joining policy-making and service-planning groups. Sarah smiled, knowing that she would have to tease out how politics played out in the organisation for Jane to make any sense of what she was seeing and prepare her for her role as a qualified nurse in the organisation in the near future.

The registration half hour in the morning was enough for Sarah to set the scene for Jane, setting out some facts about the NHS. She told her that the NHS is the largest employer in Britain and Europe, and the third largest in the world, employing about 1.3m people. Of these, up to 700,000 are nurses, midwives and health visitors. The NHS is also the single largest employer of

BME staff - 195,000 at the last count according to the Department of Health in 2005.

This contrasts with just 3 CEOs and 8 Directors of Nursing. She explained that 30% of medical students were from BME groups. Whilst it was difficult to get hold of exact numbers of BME nurses among the workforce, in 2004 the Royal College of Nursing had 59,000 overseas nurses on its books. Not only did this sector of the workforce offer nursing skills, they could also input vast cultural and emotional knowledge transferable to the heterogeneous client groups they served. Sarah explained that, despite the ethnic colour palette in the NHS workforce, the higher up you went, the whiter it became.

'The NHS management structure has been likened to Guinness,' she remarked dryly. 'Black at the bottom, white at the top.'

The experience of BME staff across the NHS had been analysed by sociologists for years, but nothing seemed to be changing. Jane was visibly surprised by what Sarah was telling her – and there was more.

'Black and minority ethnic staff get a worse deal than their white colleagues when it comes to job opportunities in the organisation,' Sarah continued. 'Although BME staff are under-represented in senior management, they are over-represented in disciplinary, grievance, bullying and harassment, and capability cases. A high proportion of BME employees are likely to be pursuing a case through an employment tribunal at any one time. A recent survey of BME staff representation in over 200 organisations in the NHS found that 16% of the workforce were BME, with just 5% executive directors, but 34% engaged in capability reviews, 44% involved in bullying and harassment cases, 31% in grievances and 29% in disciplinaries. This data suggests that BME staff experience a more challenging environment at work than their white colleagues.'

Sarah wasn't finished. She had read an RCN publication in 2005, which stated that BME nurses reported a higher incidence of bullying and harassment than their white colleagues - with over a third of BME nurses saying they had been bullied by a colleague, compared to 21 per cent of white respondents. These findings prompted RCN General Secretary Peter Carter to ask why BME nurses were contributing so much, yet receiving so little reward. In fact, BME nurses are succeeding against the odds despite the system. BME nurses are often perceived by BME patients as special advocates, fighting to defend their needs within the system on their behalf. But BME nurses confront a double challenge – discrimination amongst their patients and discrimination towards themselves. When providing services for people from BME backgrounds, the system often shies away from targeting services to areas of greatest need on the grounds of creating inequalities.

The nurses paused their deliberations as the facilitator was ready to start the course. But Jane was far more interested in talking to Sarah, and would have preferred to tease out some of these issues rather than follow the day's training.

Some of the other nurses on the course were similarly sceptical about diversity issues in the NHS, and felt that the study day and the topic they were discussing was little more than a paper exercise. They were doubtful that anything would change for either clients or staff from minority groups. Jane and Sarah had great difficulty restraining themselves during the training sessions, and couldn't wait for break periods so they could continue with the conversation they'd started that morning.

When lunchtime came, the two of them mingled with nurses from other wards in the hospital. Jane was still pondering over the information Sarah had given her earlier. She asked long-serving BME colleagues on the course whether they'd had personal experience of racism during their careers. The nurses smiled and looked at each other, waiting to see who would be brave enough to answer.

After a moment or two, Sally said, 'Some people, especially those in government and high public office, would have us believe that racism isn't an issue any more in the NHS. Politicians and unions have both worked to produce employment laws, legislation on equality and diversity, and other anti-discrimination bills to ensure fairness, equal opportunities and protection of all employees in the workplace. That is the public perception. The reality is different.'

As lunchtime wore on, the conversation around the table became lively. Three nurses from different wards in the hospital joined Jane and Sarah to eat and talk about their experiences of racism in the NHS. They all had plenty to share. It seemed that it didn't matter which hospital or community environment they worked in, their experiences were similar. One of the nurses said she was sure there was a blueprint somewhere that senior managers used to dictate behaviour, because they all acted in the same way!

The same techniques were used for discriminating against BME staff.

Nikki said she believed racism in the care profession started as early as the 1850s in the era of Mary Seacole, who spent her life developing skills in healing which she used to improve the lot of the sick. During the Crimean War, Mary followed soldiers onto the field, nursing the wounded ones back to health and being a source of comfort to the dying. Her efforts, skills and reputation rivalled Florence Nightingale's, despite Mary's additional hurdle of official indifference and prejudice towards her - for being black. Florence Nightingale was recorded in history as a legend, whilst Mary was relegated to obscurity, until about 200 years after her death, when she was recognised as the first black woman to make her mark on British public life.

'The NHS was formed soon after the Second World War,' Nikki continued, 'when there was not much money for individuals and families to pay for their health care. The organisation was hugely popular, especially as the care was free at the point of delivery. As it needed a fairly cheap but large workforce to run it, Britain invited BME personnel from around the world to come and help run the NHS and contribute to the wealth of the Nation.'

One of the other three nurses having lunch with Jane and Sarah, Joy, said it was symbolic that Great Britain had asked people from the Caribbean to come and work in the Health Service when it was first set up. Sixty years ago, hundreds of people arrived in England on the Windrush ship to perform manual jobs. They worked in the NHS and the transport services - the railways and the underground - helping to rebuild the country after the ravages of the Second World War. Yet the evidence suggests that the BME groups who arrived were treated in a second-rate way. Racism was blatant and pre-meditated, yet the attitude of the authorities was passive.

'At least now,' added Sally, 'there are laws and policies to prevent discrimination against groups of people. If you can prove that you're not getting equal opportunity or fair treatment at your workplace, you can seek recourse from the human resources department. They are obliged to investigate your allegation.'

The stimulating lunch break meant that the nurses were all fired up for the last session of the day. Empowered with new insights from their discussions, they all came up with useful ideas as to how service providers could attract and engage service users from all ethnic groups to take an interest in service planning and delivery.

Before the nurses' return to the class after lunch, Joy had concluded that the UK Racial Discrimination Act was difficult to enforce, which went some way towards explaining why the unfair treatment of BME staff in the NHS continued.

Jane was horrified. 'I thought every British citizen was law-abiding,' she said. 'I can't believe people still discriminate against ethnic minority groups when they could treat everybody equally. BME people will have to find ways of dealing with this problem.'

INSTITUTIONAL RACISM

Having been given the choice, all the nurses on the course voted to skip the afternoon tea break so that they could finish the training day early. This gave them a little more time to network, so Sarah and her group gathered at the end of the day to have a drink and finish off their debate about discrimination in their workplace. Sarah said she believed that there was institutional racism in the NHS. Its structures and processes made it possible for ethnic groups to be discriminated against, but equally very difficult for them to prove that it was happening.

Sarah also explained that communication in the NHS is generally from the top down, with channels of accountability running from the Department of Health to the Strategic Health Authorities (SHA). Information tends to flow into the chief executives of individual organisations, and from there to directors and managers and then to the rest of the staff. The rigid hierarchical management structure in the organisation and mainly white managers at the top of the management tree causes most BME nurses to assume their chances of entering management are slim. Most of them occupy the bottom tier of frontline service, and are therefore the last to receive communication about new initiatives and ideas. Sarah sketched the structure of the organisation for Jane to demonstrate how information flows to the frontline (mainly BME) staff. This is represented in the diagram on the next page.

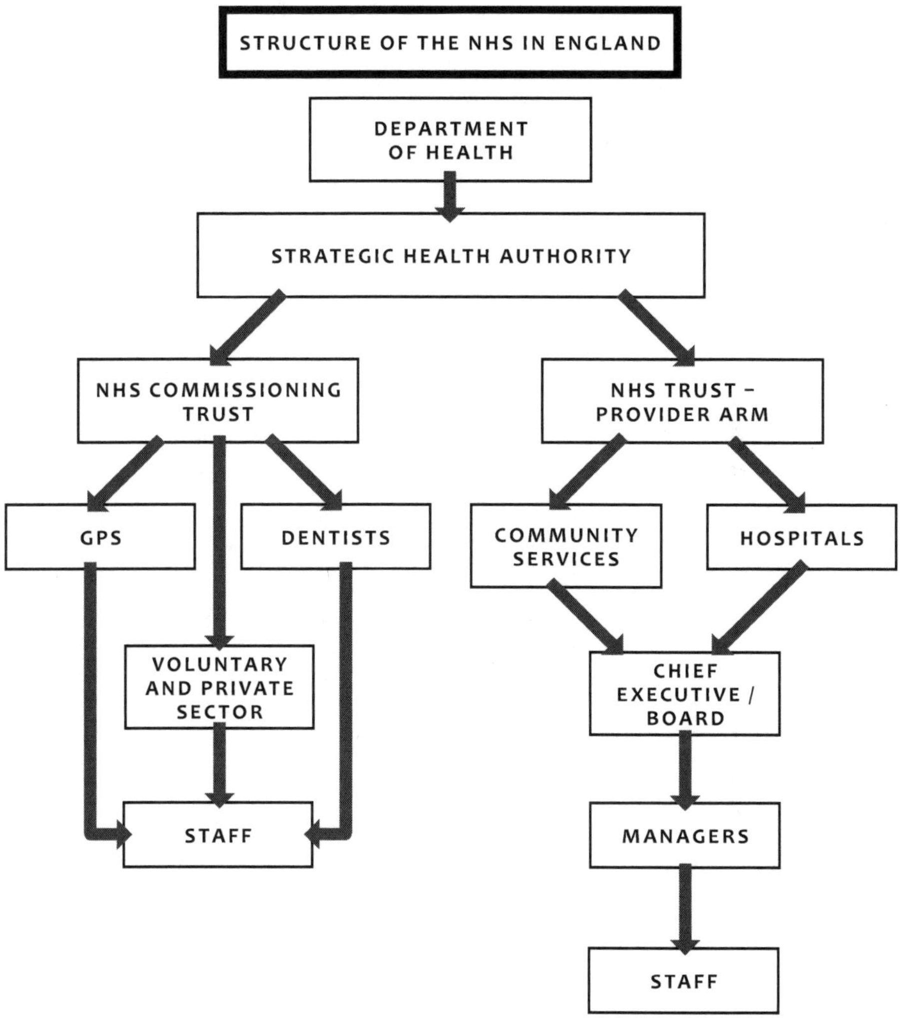
STRUCTURE OF THE NHS IN ENGLAND
DEPARTMENT OF HEALTH
STRATEGIC HEALTH AUTHORITY
NHS COMMISSIONING TRUST
NHS TRUST – PROVIDER ARM
GPS
DENTISTS
COMMUNITY SERVICES
HOSPITALS
VOLUNTARY AND PRIVATE SECTOR
CHIEF EXECUTIVE / BOARD
STAFF
MANAGERS
STAFF

Talking about discrimination at the workplace brought back memories of the past. Joy shook her head in disbelief. 'When we were celebrating the bi-centenary of the end of slavery, the media was lionising William Wilberforce as a symbol for our freedom. Slavery was abolished, but it has re-formed under a new name. Not so long ago,' she reminded her colleagues, 'the Metropolitan Police was found to be riddled with institutional racism. To be honest, that label could be applied to almost all public sector organisations, including the NHS.'

Seeing the nurses engrossed in their conversation, two of their non-BME colleagues stopped at the table on their way to buy some drinks. They didn't stay for long, though. When they realised what the subject was, they nodded here and there and then discreetly left. The subject matter was not a comfortable one. Not their fault, of course, but white staff too often feel powerless to effect change.

The discussions that day made a huge impact on Jane.

Sally asked the group to look at what happens in the entertainment world. 'Only a few from ethnic minority groups make it to the top. Black people in theatre and film get minor roles, and more often than not they play villains. Only a handful gets significant parts. We know it's not a question of talent.'

'So what is it?' Joy asked.

'Well, in music, blacks sing and white people promote and manage their talent,' Sally replied. 'I understand what usually happens is that the talent owner gets 10% of the money and the promoter gets 90%!'

They joked, but they knew it was patently unfair. Nikki said it was as if the white man had copyright over the black man's talent. And the situation was worse in sport. About a quarter of players in domestic professional football are black, but just two out of 92 league clubs have black managers in England (Chris Powell at Charlton and Paul Ince at Notts County) whilst another has just sacked its manager after an excellent spell in charge (Chris Hughton at Newcastle). Sarah, who was the only keen sportswoman among the group, said the pattern for white sports personnel was to retire from their sport and get into management, coaching or media. The black sportsman, on the other hand, disappeared into obscurity, remembered only occasionally on tribute or nostalgia programmes.

Joy replied, 'I strongly believe that racism lies beneath the discrimination and lack of opportunity that BME face, and it's rife in all spheres of life; in education, health, finance, judicial and social situations, and even in churches. BME people are missing from the boardrooms in every organisation. It's not coincidence or lack of knowledge and skills,' she persisted. 'The reality is that the ethnic minorities are actively prevented from breaking through the glass ceiling. Knowingly or unknowingly, managers and decision makers are still perpetuating this phenomenon.'

'Isn't it interesting,' Nikki commented, 'how blacks and Asians have been characterised in so many different ways: "coloured", "blacks", "Afro", "Afro-Caribbean", "Africans", "BME" and sometimes "BMAE"' (Black Minority Asian Ethnic). Joy observed drily that she would prefer it if competence rather than colour counted at work. 'If racism didn't exist', Nikki continued, 'I feel sure that between 2004 and now, the 59,000 overseas RCN-registered frontline nurses would have moved up the ladder by now - I wonder just how many have?'

The others agreed that they'd experienced discrimination and inequalities at work, and sensed that such practices were prevalent in the

NHS. Because the causes of institutional racism are multifaceted, its impact is often covert, subtle and active over a long period of time. It would take determination and commitment to eliminate this problem. People on both sides of the discrimination divide would have to work together to make a difference.

Nikki paused, then related a time when she'd applied for a job, had been shortlisted for interview, but had heard nothing more for days.

'I was at work when someone asked why I wasn't at home preparing a presentation for the interview. She said that her colleague, a non-BME who had applied for the same job, was at home doing just that. I rang the manager in charge of recruitment to find out why I hadn't been briefed about the presentation, and was told that she was just about to ring me. She would have already done so if she hadn't been pulled away to a meeting. She denied giving other candidates information days earlier and letting them have a day off to prepare for the interview. Of course,' Nikki chuckled, 'the manager wasn't aware that her "favourite" had spilt the beans and told her mates she had been given the tip-off and time off to prepare. Even so, there was nothing I could do - I might have jeopardised my chances of getting the job.'

Happily, in the end, this episode turned out well for Nikki, and both candidates were offered the job.

As the nurses parted company at the end of the evening, they exchanged ward addresses and telephone numbers, and Jane realised she'd been given some valuable insights into how the NHS operates and how it deals with its rainbow workforce.

'It's not all bad news' observed Sarah, 'there are ways to survive the system'. Her prescription for survival and to reduce the levels of stress experienced, is to understand that:

KEY POINTS

- ***Change is constant, and needs to be embraced but managed well.***
- ***Being flexible at work is essential.***
- ***Always involve all service users in service planning.***

CHAPTER 2

More Causes Than Cure

I am in earnest; I will not equivocate; I will not excuse; I will not retreat a single inch; and I will be heard.

William Garrison

ACCESS DENIED

The next day, Seacole Ward was very busy. One emergency after another kept everybody on their toes. Jane's experience from her home country stood her in good stead. She had managed similar cases with fewer resources there, so knew exactly what to do when the ward got hectic. On one level, this eased things for her mentor and trainers. However, sometimes their major task was to stop Jane from doing more than was expected of her as a nurse in training!

Sarah couldn't help noticing that Jane wasn't her usual chatty self - she seemed to just want to get on with her work. Clearly, she'd been unnerved the previous day by all the talk of discrimination and inequality. So, during their teaching and assessment time on the ward, Sarah thought she'd try to equip Jane with a few skills to protect herself and to help her advance her career.

Sarah had worked for years on several wards, often as the senior nurse with the most experience, but had never had this reflected in pay or status. On many occasions, she'd been asked to act up when the person in charge was on long-term sickness or maternity leave. But when the position became vacant and she'd applied for the post, she wasn't appointed. The excuse for this was her lack of experience - until that self-evidently couldn't be used any more. The explanation then changed to the fact that she didn't interview very well.

'When I asked managers to help me with this,' Sarah went on, 'they told me just to keep applying for jobs and going to interviews. Apparently, all I needed was practice. The irony was that, although I didn't get appointed, I was often asked to train and support the person who did get the job!'

After this had happened three or four times over five years, Sarah got fed up and decided to go and train as a psychiatric nurse. However, after two years working in mental health, she realised she was missing General Nursing.

'I knew I didn't want to go back to my old job on the General Ward,' she explained, 'so I trained as a Midwife. I've since worked in various units in hospitals and in the community. But even with over 20 years' professional experience in the NHS, I've failed to move very far up the career ladder. People working in other organisations for that length of time would be in a much better position than I am in the NHS, and it's not through lack of trying on my part!'

Joy agreed with what Sarah was saying. She said she'd watched people with fewer qualifications and far less experience than Sarah gain posts of responsibility and receive higher pay for the work they did with a lot of support from others.

This was the first time pay had been mentioned and Jane wanted to know more.

Sarah nodded. She referred to a report synthesised from nursing employment surveys for the Royal College of Nursing in 2007. This found that BME and internationally recruited nurses have to work longer to reach higher grade positions than UK white nurses -15 years to reach Senior Ward Sister, for example, compared with 11.8 years. The report also showed that nearly 60 per cent of Afro-Caribbean nurses were working in a second job compared with an average of 28 per cent of white UK nurses. As many as 70 per cent of female Afro Caribbean respondents working as staff nurses were the major bread winner compared to 44 per cent of white nurses.

Sarah, who had lived through different stages of pay structure in the organisation, tried to explain. The pay scale in nursing was very irregular before the Whitley scale was introduced; there was no consistency between job roles and remuneration. It seemed that if the bosses liked you, you received better pay and got to do the 'sexy' jobs.

Pre-Whitley Scale nurses like Mary (the other BME nurse on Seacole ward) and Sarah felt strongly that there had been blatant pay discrimination against BME staff. However, even after the introduction of the new scale, (promoted as fairer), BME staff were disappointed that inconsistencies in pay continued. The general feeling was that BME nurses were still ending up with lower pay, even if they were doing comparable or superior work to their non-BME colleagues. Individuals were allowed to negotiate their pay, and it was still possible for two people to be doing the same job, with quite different rewards.

The debate about pay inequality ran through the command structure and, in the 1980s, the pay structure was changed once again, this time to Grading. In this system, qualified nurses started on Grade D and could go up to H or I. Sarah pointed out that during this period about 80% of BME nurses were on D grade, with 20% on E. White nurses, on the other hand, were on higher grades, with 80% on E and the top 20% on F.

'There were hundreds of unsuccessful appeals from BME nurses about their low pay,' Sarah recalled. 'Apart from the moral obligation of employers to give equal pay to all groups of staff in order to build a successful business, they were also obliged to cultivate an atmosphere of creativity with high productivity. Valuing diversity and treating all staff groups equally was supposed to achieve that goal. In fact, this pay scale approach produced the opposite, poisoning working relationships among the different ethnic groups on the wards.'

The current pay structure is Agenda For Change (AFC). Like its predecessors, it has its advantages and disadvantages. Its intention was for the job role to be graded, rather than the person in the role. This would ensure that all personnel in different organisations received the same pay for the same role and responsibility. AFC is banded from 2 to 9, and studies have found that most BME nurses are concentrated at bands 3 to 5. This pay structure has succeeded in bringing an improvement in fairness, but there have been cases where individuals have been able to negotiate higher banding or points for the same job role than their colleagues. Sarah added that the RCN and other government bodies were working towards improving visible diversity in leadership roles in response to the increasing diversity within nursing. There is now a strong call to include, listen to, care for and respect nurses from diverse backgrounds. This links with a recognition that a diverse workforce is necessary to meet local health needs.

'But,' Sarah pointed out, 'because BME staff are over-represented in routine and semi-routine jobs, they're more likely to be made redundant when there is any restructuring or merger of services in NHS organisations - unless, the pay-off is substantial, where they cease to be the first choice.'

Jane was incensed. 'I can't believe these things have been allowed to go on for so long,' she muttered. 'I'll certainly be making my voice heard when I'm a fully fledged nurse.'

But Mary shook her head. 'Let me give you a piece of free advice, Jane. As a BME, if you decide to challenge some of these injustices, you should be careful because it might come back to bite you. There's a fair (or should that be, unfair) chance that after you've challenged a decision, your job could be vulnerable in any restructuring or merger of services. Even if your post is vital to the success of the organisation, it's likely to be re-configured, rebranded and advertised. Your successor, likely to have been hand-picked, will be appointed to the post and there'll be absolutely nothing you can do about it.'

MIND THE GAP

Overhearing this, Sarah nodded to herself. The most common barrier to BME staff progression is withholding opportunities to perform at their level of expertise. It's as if they are not trusted to perform at that level and, if they do get the chance, it's generally because no one else could be found, or because they're needed to step-up temporarily in someone's absence. Many BME staff say they feel that, whenever they are given a chance, they feel under scrutiny.

They don't routinely get feedback for a job well done. Sarah decided to pass on to Jane how to overcome this particular hurdle.

'After all,' she laughed, 'I've had enough practice at breaking the code! What you have to do is make people aware that you are conspicuously capable of doing your work and doing it well. BME staff need to get into the habit of asking about job opportunities, and challenging perceptions, rather than colluding with discriminatory practices by saying nothing. I once worked with a nurse who did all of these things. She was a BME nurse working with a non-BME in the same department. One day the manager of the unit left unexpectedly and cover was needed. Replacing a member of staff is quite a lengthy process, especially at management level. So, while the organisation went in search of a replacement, the non-BME staff member was asked to step into the role. She had a good six-month run of managing the unit till the new manager arrived. For some reason, the newly appointed manager didn't stay in the job, and left in less than two years. Again, the non-BME staff member was asked to step in. But this time, my BME colleague challenged the decision and said it was her time to deputise as a manager.'

Jane was all ears. 'What happened?' she asked.

Sarah shrugged. 'Sadly, rather than allow her to have a go, they left the position vacant until another new recruit was appointed. But it was worthwhile, because at least she made people aware that she existed and wanted to be treated fairly.'

Jane nodded. Clearly she was going to have to be proactive and ask for opportunities to learn, practise and progress in her area of work.

One day in the staff canteen, Nikki met up with Sarah and Jane, and they caught up with each other's news and general hospital gossip. Then Jane directed the conversation back to equality and diversity among staff in the NHS. It's an emotive subject that affects most BME staff, and they enjoy being able to talk about it. It's how they support each other.

Nikki described how, a few years before, she had successfully applied for a specialist role on the ward where she worked. Before she had properly taken it up, a new, non-BME nurse joined her team, who coveted the role Nikki had just been appointed to. Without any explanation, the new nurse on the ward was assigned to the specialist role.

'I finally mustered up the courage to ask Management what was going on,' she recalled. 'I wanted to know why I was being given general nursing duties while my colleague had been given the specialist role that I should have been doing. It turned out that managers were hoping I wouldn't say anything about the swap over, asking me if I wanted to continue with the role I was already doing. Apparently, on arrival on the ward, the new nurse had decided she wanted the specialist role, and had spoken to the managers about it. The ward sister had agreed that the new girl could have the job, even though I'd interviewed successfully for it!' Nikki looked indignant, 'I told them I didn't want to carry on in my old role, and asked for the specialist nurse role, the role I'd been appointed to. You see, Jane', Nikki insisted, 'the trick is to be openly competent in what you do, and insist on having your voice heard. That's how these inequalities will stop. If more people stood up and did that, recruitment processes would become colour-blind.'

'BME staff are successful at getting promotion when they go for jobs that white nurses aren't too keen on', Sarah explained. 'This applies to doctors' posts as well. The "Cinderella" jobs – the ones that are heavy, demanding and stressful - usually attract little interest from non-BME groups. These jobs are for BME employees. I remember a day when the ward upstairs had an acute shortage of staff, so I was asked to cover a shift. Many of the people who came to the ward that day did a double take. They asked me at the nurses' station to find the person in charge for them. The look on their faces when I told them I was the one in charge! Some were brazen enough to ask me twice, but to be honest, I'm so used to being patronised by patients and colleagues that I took no notice and simply said again, "It's me. I'm in charge of the ward"'

The late shift on Thursday saw Sarah and Jane teamed up again. Sarah wasn't feeling well but managed to finish the shift. The next day Sarah was still off and Jane felt a little apprehensive about how the day would turn out in support terms. Inside there was a palpable fear of working with someone new, who might be less sympathetic. As a trainee, Jane had to work under supervision. Looking around that day, there was no other BME on duty apart from her. Word came that she was to work with Nurse Molly White. Jane had seen Molly a few times on the ward but had not spoken to her so didn't know how she would relate to her. Jane was relieved when Molly approached, greeted her warmly and told her about the work plan for that morning. Molly was chatty, genuinely interested in Jane's experiences and happy to share her own.

Jane and Molly shared their break together talking all the while - and Jane learnt new ways of doing the nursing duties that day. Before the end of the day Molly told Jane she could come to her if she needed help with anything. By the end of the shift Jane was in a great mood, inspired by her positive experience of working with a non-BME. Molly had been generous with her time and tuition. On her way home Jane reflected that with people like Molly and the determination of BME staff, equality of opportunity could be achieved in the NHS.

UNSEEN, UNHEARD, UNDERVALUED

The following Monday morning, Sarah and Jane were back on duty. The ward was busy with a number of critically ill patients. There were lots to do and Sarah was grateful for trainee Jane's previous experience which enabled her to care for high-dependency patients with minimum supervision. In fact, Jane's residual knowledge saved the day. Jane was competent enough to carry out some of the procedures that were usually done by junior doctors on the ward.

This was borne out in practice. The medical consultant was due to do a ward round to review his patients. Jane and Sarah had been working flat out without a break when the retinue of consultant and his team of junior doctors arrived on the ward. On cue, as the doctors arrived at Nurse James' and Student Nurse Oladejide's bay, Sister McLaughlin sprang out of her office ready to do the ward round with the doctors.

The team moved in a stately fashion around the ward with the Consultant directing his questions about the patients to the Sister. The problem was, Sister McLaughlin had been in her office all morning, without any direct involvement in the care given to any of the patients.

Jane watched as the Consultant spoke to the Sister, who in turn asked Sarah for the answers, before feeding them back to the Consultant.

It went something like this:

Consultant: 'How is Mr Smith doing on his new medication?'

Sister: 'Nurse James, how is Mr Smith doing on his new medication? '

Sarah:	'Mr Smith is responding well. His blood pressure is coming down and his breathing has improved. He doesn't need the oxygen mask when he's mobile.'
Sister:	'He's responding well. His blood pressure is coming down, his breathing has improved, and he doesn't need the oxygen mask when he's mobile.'

This was replicated for each of the eight patients on Sarah's side of the ward. The only time Sarah spoke directly to the Consultant was when her answer was too complicated for Sister McLaughlin to pass on. During this process Sarah and Jane were ignored, almost as if they were invisible.

Sister McLaughlin was on top of the world as she went from patient to patient with the ward round party. She conversed freely with the Consultant, even interrupting him on occasions when he was teaching the junior doctors.

'If I didn't know better,' Sarah quipped later, 'I'd have thought Sister didn't want the consultant to leave!'

The ward round was Jane's first on Seacole. Seeing her looking bemused, Sarah said, 'Let me explain what went on this morning. Remember the blueprint that was mentioned on the training day - the invisible code, manifesto if you like, that seems to govern the behaviour of the consultants, and managers in the Health Service? Well, that code says that consultants can choose not to speak to BME nurses, but they can communicate with them through the white ones.'

Jane's jaw dropped in disbelief. She was genuinely shocked.

Sarah laughed. 'I'm joking - but the way some people behave in this organisation, you could easily believe that they are working to a code like that! My father told me that, in the past, white people believed the black man was inferior, less intelligent than them. If you ask people now, they will not admit to that, but their actions speak for them. Generally, senior doctors will talk only to certain types of nurses on the ward - unless the doctor himself is black, which is rare.'

Jane shook her head, remembering how something similar had happened to her last week when she was with a patient, and a relative had wanted to enquire after the patient's progress.

'She asked the nurse in the next bay when I was right there! I mean, the relative saw me caring for the patient. The nurse in the other bay assumed I wasn't around and came to look for me so that I could talk to the relative – after all, this wasn't her patient. How was she supposed to know what the situation was? I told the other nurse that the relative had seen me in the bay but chose to ask someone else. Anyway, we ended up having a three-way conversation. I thought it was strange at the time, but didn't fully understand what was going on. Now I do.'

By the time the ward round was over, the consultant and his team of admirers had gone, the patients were comfortable, and the excitable sister had slipped back into her office, it was mid-morning.

'I could kill for a cup of tea,' grinned Sarah and Jane agreed that they needed a break.

Just as they were on their way to ask their colleagues to cover for them, Sister McLaughlin emerged from her office and informed them that they had to cover Nurse Julie as she'd been asked to attend a meeting on Sister's behalf. The upshot of this was that Sarah and Jane would miss their tea break, and their workload had doubled.

Sarah cast a meaningful glance in Jane's direction. Julie was clearly the chosen one of the ward – the one being groomed. On Sister's invitation, she'd actively joined in the ward round – 'It'll be a good learning and networking opportunity for you.' Because she hadn't finished her work caring for the patients in her bay, Sarah and Jane would have to bear the brunt of the workload so that she could attend the strategic meeting for Sister.

Even though all senior nurses were supposed to take it in turns to attend these meetings, Julie seemed to be the only one who ever went. Sarah was the most senior nurse on the ward, and was asked to deputise for Sister when there were heavy cases or difficulties. She could rightfully expect to be given the opportunity to attend some of the meetings where staff from all three medical wards came together with senior managers and consultants to discuss patient issues and schedules.

'No one else is ever given the chance to attend,' Sarah complained, once she and Jane were out of range of Sister McLaughlin. 'In fact, we don't even know when the meetings are due to happen. Sister used to announce the dates at our team meetings, but she's stopped doing that for some reason.'

Jane noticed the disappointment in Sarah's eyes and tried to cheer her. 'Don't worry,' she smiled. 'Time goes quicker when you're busy. We'll get finished in no time. Then we can have our break.'

With that, the two nurses got on with seeing to Julie's patients, but Jane caught Sarah say under her breath, 'It's happening all over again.'

'What's it?' Jane asked.

Sarah was silent for a moment. Then, in a low voice she said, 'Do you remember my telling you the other day that I've recently come back into general nursing after broadening my CV in other fields? Well, after a year on this ward, the Sister in charge left and I was asked to act up until a successor was found. To save money, replacing the Ward Sister was delayed for six months, but that was my opening, and everybody said how good I was at the job. But when the time came to appoint permanently, I didn't get it! Sister McLaughlin was appointed. She had recently qualified as a registered nurse and was a band 5. I was a band 6, but she was given the promotion to band 7.'

She paused.

'I was coerced into feedback from my interview,' she said finally. 'I say "coerced" because by then I was resigned to the fact that I didn't get the job because I was black. It's an obvious conclusion to draw because I had been successfully running the ward the day before the interview, and I thought I'd performed well at the interview. This wouldn't happen to a white nurse. I was told at the feedback session that I was an inch away from the mark. The person who got the job apparently gave the right answers so they had to appoint her. What followed was the last straw. I was told that the panel realised the new Sister didn't have the experience of running a critical medical ward like this, so they asked me to train her on the job! Dumbfounded, I responded, "I'm sorry?" The Manager realised what she'd said, and quickly changed the word "train" to "assist", explaining that the new Sister would need a lot of support from me.'

Jane was flabbergasted. 'Let me get this straight,' she said. 'You were a band 6 with experience and a track record proving that you could do the job, but you weren't offered it. Yet a newly-qualified nurse with no experience got the post, jumping from band 5 to 7, and you had to train - sorry, "support" - her. So she got to learn the job from the top! I thought people worked up from the bottom!'

Sarah answered ruefully, 'I'm afraid not. That opportunity was reserved for non-BME only.'

Jane didn't know what else to say, so she started to laugh, shaking her head in disbelief.

'It's not a laughing matter,' insisted Sarah. 'I've been summoned to meetings with senior managers where I've had to respond to charges made by Sister against me that I'm not helping her do her job! In the early days when the ward got very busy, she'd go into her office and cry.'

'Why?' Jane asked, incredulously.

Sarah shrugged. 'Stress. I suppose she just wasn't coping. She eventually went off sick for a few weeks before coming back for more of the same.'

'So what happened?' Jane wanted to know. 'How did you cope with such an awkward situation?'

'Not very well,' Sarah replied, 'Sister McLaughlin had the keys to the drugs cabinet and the ward, and took the plaudits as the boss, and I made all the tough decisions and managed the day-to-day activity. I did the work, she got the kudos.'

'Why didn't you just leave?'

Sarah gave another resigned shrug. 'I have a mortgage to pay and this hospital is near home, so I don't have far to travel to work. That's the only reason I'm still here. But I have stop thinking about it. These days I do the bare minimum to get through the day, then go home.'

'Your patients aren't getting the best of you, then,' Jane remarked.

'And whose fault's that?' was the terse response.

Jane sighed. 'It's not fair. Something has to be done to stop all this.'

Time flew. The shift was soon over. Jane and Sarah had a couple of well-deserved days off. The following Monday, they were both back at work. Later in the day they reserved some time to go through the documentation to record Jane's progress in adapting to nursing in England. Just before lunch, the nurses took leave to go through the paperwork they had to complete for the supervising University.

Jane was doing well on the Adaptation Course and it was easy for Sarah to complete the assessment book.

The next step was for Jane to take it to the University for her lecturers to officially certificate her. Sarah's advice was, 'Once you decide what it is you want to do, specialise in it and be consistently good at doing it.'

As they walked back to the ward, she told Jane that she could be successful in her nursing career. Change was happening – but it was happening slowly.

The most important thing was to:

KEY POINTS

- ***Be passionate about your work and do it well.***
- ***Keep up with changes – re-invent yourself if you have to.***
- ***Ask for the pay that matches your expertise.***

CHAPTER 3

Double Standards

If you are distressed by anything external, the pain is not due to the thing itself, but to your estimate of it; and this you have the power to revoke at any moment.

Marcus Aurelius

GROOMING FOR SUCCESS

Sarah told Jane that some nurses are selected and groomed for promotion by people in positions of power. These nurses are supplied with all the information and training necessary to climb up the ladder. They are afforded the opportunity to practise, to shadow and to learn their trade. Unsurprisingly, they step into the shoes of the top people. In the main, these are not nurses from BME backgrounds.

'In every job,' Sarah said, 'there are implicit and explicit procedures and rituals. If you are privy to these trade secrets, of course you'll do well. But history shows that BME are not usually given these opportunities. BME nurses are less likely to be given the opportunity to act up in a job, or go on secondment and later successfully apply for the job.

'It's common practice in the NHS for senior managers to invite people to apply for positions, and the invitees are usually the ones groomed! If a manager tells someone to apply for a job, the chances are high that they will be successful at securing the job.'

Jane was finding it increasingly difficult to believe her ears. 'But I thought the NHS was an equal opportunities employer. How can this happen?'

'The NHS is an equal opportunities employer on paper,' Sarah replied. 'Talk to the BME nurses and you'll soon find out the truth. More than nine out of ten of BME staff would say they have experienced discrimination of some sort in the organisation. There are ways of ignoring statutory guidelines and not getting caught, especially when no one is monitoring organisations for compliance. When a job is advertised what you have to do, Jane, is discreetly investigate whether someone's name has been pencilled in for that job. If it has, you will be wasting your time applying, and by putting in an application you are simply helping people to tick boxes to say that they have advertised and identified the right person for the job.'

Jane was curious. 'But how can you tell if a job is sewn up before it's advertised?'

Sarah laughed. 'It comes with experience. You can't learn everything in one day. Once you start working, you'll soon get to recognise the person who's being groomed for promotion. They're very easy to spot - a little like the teacher's pet at school. These nurses get every shift they want, they get weekends, seasonal breaks off – they always get first bite of the cherry.

'And they can always supply reasons - medical certificates for instance - why they are unable to do the hard work. The mistakes they make are unavoidable, because someone else was at error first and caused the chain of events. If the mistake does fall into the public domain, the incident will be written off as a learning experience. This doesn't mean that your mistakes will be treated in the same way,' she warned. 'If you do anything wrong, Jane, you'll find yourself at home writing your statement and talking to your union before you know it.

'There are perks that accompany being a manager's pet. Extra time off for doing work for the boss - or alibis made available which means that they can say that they are too busy to support the ward team. It's difficult to know what they're up to most of the time, off sick or on holiday on business or on personal retreat. They even get time off to bury deceased pets, while the non-groomed often have to fight to get time off to bury their relatives! They get on like a house on fire with the bosses, because it won't be long before they are invited to join the club. Nurses like that have access to inside information, sometimes about other managers. They are a great source of gossip. People know these practices go on but no one says anything, because of a fear of losing their jobs'.

Even though Sarah was relatively sanguine about this, Jane wasn't happy. She was a senior nurse back home. She knew she had the experience and knowledge to rise to the level she'd been performing at there, and beyond if she worked hard. The scenario Sarah described worried her and she began to wonder if she'd done the right thing in joining the NHS.

OFFICE ETIQUETTE

Jane went to the University to meet with her lecturer and go through her portfolio, which was a record of how she was progressing on the ward. She was now halfway through the course, and her reports were excellent. Jane returned to the ward in jubilant mood to celebrate her good news with Sarah.

As she walked in, she met some of her nursing colleagues at the nurses' station talking with the Ward Clerk, Ms Woodward. Ms Woodward was someone to be obeyed at all times if you wanted a stress-free day at work. Jane said hello to her mates, but none of them responded. There seemed to be a group fascination with the clock on the wall.

On the ward, Jane found Sarah working assiduously, talking to her patients, and waited for an opportune moment to pass on the good news she'd received from her lecturer. Sarah was delighted, and said she would celebrate with her at break time.

'Can I ask you a question?' Jane asked. 'I arrived and said hello to the girls at the front just now, and no one responded. Instead they all looked at the clock. Why is that? This has happened before. I used to think they must be very busy or hadn't heard me, but then someone else would come in and they'd respond heartily - especially on a Monday when they would catch up on the weekend's activities. If they're being selective about who they relate to at work, that's not building a team. It's really uncomfortable to be ignored while everybody else is deep in conversation.'

Sarah shook her head. 'Take no notice,' she sighed. 'They need to be trained in public relations. Most of them will be taking short breaks, cigarette breaks, and catching up on the latest gossip, but won't be prioritising working. I know I'd never get away with that, so what do I do? I work. When someone looks at the clock when you arrive, it means they're checking your arrival time, noticing that you're late. Nurse Webb always looks at the clock when I come in to work, even when I'm on time. She's the ward timekeeper, despite never finishing the work she's allocated. You'd be surprised. If it ever became an issue, she'd have all the data ready – every date, time and shift when you came to work late.'

'Wow!' Jane replied, eyebrows raised. 'Sounds as if we haven't just got nurses on the ward - we've got covert agents, too.'

Sarah grinned. 'Of course, don't forget, Britain won the Cold War!'

'You know, sometimes,' Jane went on, 'I meet my ward colleagues outside of the hospital, and you'd think they don't know me. Even if they could pronounce my name, they can't remember it. But I know all of them and their names.' There was real anger in her voice now. 'Where I come from, it's very rude not to acknowledge someone when they greet you. Wouldn't it be better if they said hello and then asked me why I was late? How can you not talk to somebody, but keep a record of their movements as evidence for the prosecution?'

As Sarah and Jane worked through the rest of the shift, Jane asked more questions about the arcane behaviour of her colleagues.

'Now that we're cracking the code,' she persisted, 'what does it mean when you speak and people look up and roll their eyes upwards? I see them do that during handover sometimes, when dealing with routine questions.'

Sarah explained, 'Looking up, rolling eyes upwards, a head shake - these can mean, "Unbelievable", "Liar", or it might be a way to show off, make fun of you or discredit you. I wouldn't worry about it. It happens too often to be tackled each time. It's best to ignore it and get on with your work. If it really bothers you, you could have a word with the people involved and tell them how their gestures and remarks make you feel. But be ready for the fallout, because once you confront people, they label you. You might be called touchy, aggressive, sensitive, and weird. Once you challenge something you're noticed, your card is marked, exacerbating the situation. Then you find yourself excluded from the clique. Sometimes it's much better just to keep quiet rather than say anything.' She smiled. 'You need to try and rise above these things, Jane. They're really not important. I say hello to people when I see them, and if they choose not to respond, I don't bother the next time. When people are ready to talk, I'll talk to them. If not, well, we're here to work anyway.

'This ward is notorious for its cliques - if you're not in the inner circle, people are reluctant to talk to you. That's not very heart-warming I know, but give it time and you will make friends, with colleagues on this ward or on others. If someone on this ward takes a liking to you, go with the flow. But be observant, watch what people are doing and do the same, but remember that your actions, whilst identical to your colleagues', could get you into trouble. My advice is, keep on top of your game and be vigilant. Don't give people any excuse to discriminate against you. You will need to be self-contained as an individual as well as integrated into a team – defend your personal space and only allow people in who you trust.'

Jane was beginning to realise that working in the NHS wasn't as easy as people thought. She told Sarah how happy her family back home were that she was working in a British hospital.

'It's not all bad,' Sarah countered, 'especially on pay day at the end of the month. It tends to anaesthetise the hardship you had to go through to get your money.'

The following week on one of the early shifts, a consultant was looking for one of his patients' blood results in vain. It wasn't his practice to speak to Jane, but because he needed the results he called her to locate them for him. Jane, however, had already asked the assistant on the ward to go and collect the results, without success. Frowning, she remembered that she had asked the ward clerk to do other tasks for her as well, but had been blanked.

The consultant was annoyed that the blood results weren't on the ward before he arrived, and Jane got into trouble even though she had delegated that task to someone else. Hearing about this, Sarah said she could feel another masterclass coming on!

'Sometimes even the junior staff find it difficult to take orders from BME staff,' she said. 'A BME might ask an assistant to do something, and they will still go and check with somebody, usually a white person (often junior to the BME who sent them!) before they feel comfortable complying. The ward assistants, ward clerks and secretaries will monitor BME staff like hawks, and will be the first to blow the whistle if there is the suggestion of any wrongdoing by a BME.'

TRIBAL

Sarah, who was inherently wise and tried to bring balance to every situation, observed that it was sometimes a matter of culture.

'Many of us come from different countries and do things differently. You like to bring in your jolloff rice for lunch. Someone else might bring in canned soup, sandwiches or pre-packed foods to microwave. People might be keen to see, smell and even taste your food because it's exotic. Some are genuinely interested, whilst others may have different motives for monitoring what culturally diverse food is coming into the workplace.'

'It must be the same with "culturally diverse" names,' Jane remarked. 'When my friend came to see where I worked recently, she was surprised to hear people calling me "Jane". I had to explain to her that they couldn't be bothered to learn my name, Adenike Oladejide, so they asked me to answer to the name "Jane" because that's what the last part of my surname sounds like. I had to adjust to their needs rather than the other way around.'

'Oh, yeah!' laughed Sarah. 'I've known people who changed their original names to Western ones to get jobs! We call that getting a passport name'.

'Well, that's just plain rude,' Jane said. 'I am new to the country but I'm doing my best with McLaughlin and O'Callaghan and Cunningham!'

Sarah said that what really got under her skin was accent-based differentiation. People from Africa and the Caribbean were treated differently because of the way they spoke. 'People make judgements about you as soon as you open your mouth,' she commented. 'They don't listen to you properly, because they've made up their minds in advance that they can't understand what you're saying. In contrast, BME staff try to understand all kinds of accents – Brummie, Scouse, Geordie and even those strange Scottish brogues!'

As a newcomer to the ward, Jane said that sometimes she hadn't realised her colleagues were speaking English when they spoke to her. She'd had to ask someone to 'translate' for her! Some of her colleagues had also described her as "loud" because she liked to dress and talk in a certain way.

'I think colour in clothing and in appearance generally adds a touch of vibrancy. Some of my colleagues wish I'd change and be like them, to "tone things down"! But I like the way I am. That is what diversity is all about - embracing each other's idiosyncrasies.'

'I'm glad we get on,' Sarah smiled. 'Sometimes, Africans and West Indians don't. The media describe black inter-racial disputes as "black on black" crime. There's a tendency to characterise this as a kind of tribal war going on between the two groups of people - which of course is bad news for both.'

'I don't understand,' Jane frowned. 'You'd have thought they would get on since they share the same experience.'

'You must have heard the saying, "A divided kingdom will not stand",' Sarah replied.

'I think West Indians haven't really forgiven Africans for selling them to the white man all those centuries ago,' Jane continued. 'The West Indians consider themselves more westernised than the Africans, and the Africans think they have their own heritage and don't have to adopt another's.'

'That's one of the reasons why BME are struggling in many areas of life. They don't have a strong, united voice in Society,' Sarah shrugged. 'Some of the BME staff, in their quest to be accepted, have resorted to selling their colleagues out - to management, offering to spy on their fellow BME to win approbation. They are known as "coconuts" - black on the outside but white inside. Because of their eagerness to be accepted in the inner circle they have been prepared to betray their colleagues for tiny rewards', she added, 'but it's a sad state of affairs. Until all BME staff realise that they have a common heritage and a shared interest in standing up against inequality, nothing much will change. When we fight each other, all we do is give the reactionaries and bigots more reason to keep us beneath the glass ceiling.

'The way I see it,' Sarah concluded, 'is that all BME staff possess a map telling them where the treasure of equal opportunity lies, but until they unearth the treasure chest, they can't share the wonderful gold of liberty, equality and fraternity with each other'.

'I see it this way,' Jane replied. 'All BME people are in a house together. The house is on fire, but instead of collectively trying to put the fire out, they're squabbling over the house contents. It's a self-destructive strategy, because in the meantime, the house will burn to the ground. The priority should be to put out the fire and then they can worry about the contents.

'What BME staff should do,' she said thoughtfully, 'is to stop fighting each other and form mutually supportive networks. Our non-BME colleagues are brilliant at networking. There is a cohort of managers from the same ethnic background in the organisation to teach them the trade. There are very few BME managers and the upper slopes of management in the NHS are white-tipped. BME staff should start supporting each other if they're going to move forward together. That means new rules in a new game - one that is based around the team rather than individual performance.

'To win that game', Jane said, 'the team needs to:'

KEY POINTS

- ***Make their voices heard.***
- ***Be more politically aware.***
- ***Read the writing on the wall.***

Section Two

Care Profession Casualties - The New Game

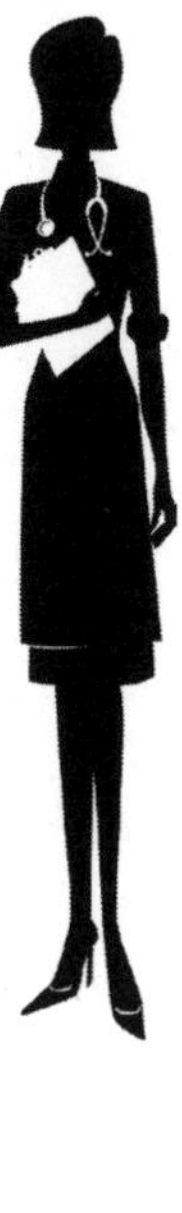

CHAPTER 4

The Rules Have Changed

The greatest obstacle
to discovery is not ignorance- it is
the illusion of knowledge.

Daniel Boorstin

NO JOB SECURITY, HIGH DEBT

Summer had arrived. It was lighter in the mornings and the evenings seemed to stretch out into the distance. Jane was four months into her training and doing well. She couldn't wait to qualify, start working and earn better money. Sarah, meanwhile, was doing all she could to equip Jane for her career in the NHS. She knew her student wouldn't have any problems qualifying. The gaps in her knowledge lay in understanding the political infrastructure and some of the precepts that supported it. These were the invisible rules of work.

Sarah was passionate about change. She and her generation had suffered institutional discrimination in the NHS for years and it was time for the new guard to advance without these unnecessary shackles. The Government was now actively addressing racism in the NHS and legislation, different strategies and new frameworks were emerging to support that aspiration. But the BME had to play their part in this process, to add their determination and strength to the wheel to turn it faster.

Sarah had a friend, Judith, who had retired from the NHS. She had climbed from the foothills to one of the higher basecamps in the lee of the pinnacle of the NHS. She had been heading towards a Director's role when restructuring within the organisation had led to her being made redundant. Sarah knew that here was an insider, someone who knew the rules and how to play the game. It was time to talk to Judith.

Judith had kept in contact with some of her ex-colleagues, including people in the Department of Health, so she was up to date with what was happening in the NHS - more so than some people in the organisation. Whenever Sarah visited her, she was alerted to plans in the health pipeline. Judith's sources were current – and accurate.

'We'll go and see Judith,' Sarah said to Jane decisively. 'She'll help. She's bound to know inside information about how we can make our ideas work in practice. She'll be a huge asset to us, I'm sure. We've got a day off on Wednesday. I'll speak to her and see if we can go then.'

When Wednesday arrived, Judith was ready for them, with more than tea and cakes on offer. She'd gathered together a pile of documents, strategies, reports and white papers ready to share with the girls.

Judith launched the informal symposium with an unsettling statement: 'There is no job security any more – regardless of whether you are black or white.

'The global economic melt down and its outworking in Britain has changed the way business operates,' she explained. 'Especially in the public sector where the writing is on the wall. However, the NHS is close to people's hearts in this country, and they'll fight to preserve it. In the meantime, economic turbulence has holed the ship beneath the waterline – money is flowing out of the system like water and the politicians and administrators are bailing out excess baggage as fast as HMS NHS slips downwards. That surplus weight might include the likes of you and I – but it could also include borderline cancer victims, people who inflict illness on themselves like heavy smokers and drinkers and whole layers of the senior management structure. The line that GP-run local NHS Trusts will return the service back to the patients is a good PR story. But it's really about the money. It's nothing new,' Judith continued. 'We've seen it all before. I just hope we've learnt from history and can apply those lessons to the present situation. Then we'll survive and even move forward.

'Throughout previous recessions – even when times were very perilous indeed in the Eighties, the NHS was immune from drastic cuts as it held a sacrosanct position in the Nation's affections. This time, however, it is being asked to make major efficiency savings and absorb fundamental reorganisation that will have profound implications for the employment structure of the organisation. Some nurses are calling it "cuts through the back door". With the passing of job security, a major recession biting hard, and the presence of widespread institutional discrimination I fear for those of our people who are not politically astute and ready to defend their rights.'

The light was dawning for Jane. 'Does this mean that the recession will place BME staff more in danger of losing jobs and opportunities? And widen the cultural/racial opportunity gap?' She asked.

Sarah looked pensive. 'Only time will tell, I suppose. But we're not going to wait for it to start happening. That's why we're here - to find out how we keep our jobs and how to stay ahead of the game.

'What seems to be happening,' she went on, thinking aloud, 'is that extraordinary external forces are widening existing institutional cracks to create major faultlines in the economy and in people's lives. The credit crunch, job losses, massive cuts in public services and increased taxation, in addition to the high cost of living, will hurt millions of people, especially the already under-privileged BME. Many professionals, including nurses face seeing their living standards and their years of training swallowed up by economic stringencies. Everything we are witnessing at present is threatening to undermine the progress that we have made as a BME Community.'

Judith looked directly at the two of them. 'It's time for you nurses to start thinking outside the box, and to start looking outside it as well. You'll have to be creative in your thinking to anticipate and subvert the institutional pressures being brought to bear on you. What will happen if the decision-makers announce restructuring or merger strategies to save money? There's no guarantee any of you will retain your jobs. At best you might be redeployed to a different department, not of your choice. You will have a simple decision to make: to take it or leave it.'

Jane was horrified. 'That's outrageous!' she exclaimed.

'This is how it works.' Judith explained, 'If you are lucky enough not to go through restructuring, vacancies will be frozen and the fortunate few who remain in employment will be stretched thinly to cover the work.' Yes, you know the phrase: "Work differently and work smartly."'

'But is that possible?' Jane asked. 'Can the managers make any one they choose do two people's jobs?'

'I think they'll make us do more than that,' Sarah replied. 'You'll be made to feel as if you're lucky to be employed, so if your boss says "jump" you'll be expected to answer, "what is the current high jump record?" '

Jane looked at Judith. 'So is this the time to be asking for equal rights? In a credit crunch, any abrasive noise you make will be turned into an opportunity to get rid of you.'

'That's the easy option,' Sarah sighed, 'shut up and put up. Most BME will go along with that as they have mortgages and other debts, and they need to be in jobs with constant running money attached. This is not acceptable because mortgages and debts are always with us and in any case people are deferring retirement.'

'But some of my friends who are businessmen,' interjected Judith, 'define having a job as being "just over broke". There are people with regular monthly paid jobs who are an unlucky bet away from being insolvent. Given that it's becoming more difficult at present to keep your nose above the water economically, it's more important than ever before to have an independent assessment of your career in order to discover routes out of this trap. There are people who can help you if you're interested.'

TECHNOLOGY AND INFORMATION SUPER HIGHWAY

Judith told her small audience that this was a completely new era. Nursing had changed a lot from when she was working in it, and the way nursing care was provided these days was a whole new ball game.

'Nursing has become separated from caring,' she said. 'A nurse will give an injection and a carer will do the bed baths and feeding. But the nurse is blamed when the patient fails to thrive through poor care - even though the nurse doesn't manage the carer. Nurses and carers work for different organisations which makes no sense. However, that's a conversation for another day. Roles in hospital have been redefined. The who, what and how of nursing evolve constantly. This reappraisal of roles is necessary because of changing community needs, new technology and ever-diminishing resources.

'There has been a revolution in information technology, and how it affects society. Patient information and care is available for staff to access at the click of a button. That part of it is incredibly exciting. There is new information on the Internet continually, and it's important for professionals to keep up to date.'

Sarah and Jane were so engrossed in what Judith was saying that their tea went cold in the cups. Judith paused to make a fresh pot and then picked up from where she'd left off.

'How much of your work is on computer?' she asked.

The two nurses said that most of it was. The work was generated, allocated and evaluated on computer, enabling managers to see instantly how much work was being done and by whom. Judith was gratified to hear that their IT skills were good.

'As I talk to people from different NHS organisations,' she said, 'I realise that some nurses are really struggling in that area. They have no computer skills and seem unwilling to learn. This will definitely be a barrier to progression in the future. Being proficient in IT defines you as a modern nurse and is one of the ways to ensure you keep your job. No professional can afford to be computer illiterate.'

HIGH QUALITY SERVICE, LOW COST DELIVERY

Judith sipped her tea thoughtfully. 'Right,' she said, 'we've established that any information you need is now readily available on the Internet. That means that all your patients have got access to the same information as the professionals. Gone are the days when doctors knew best and patients did as they were told. We have witnessed the arrival of the "expert patient" - someone who knows more about their illness and managing it than the medical professionals! Knowledge of current best practice, the latest research and new work on treatment and the management of most medical conditions are essential if you want to be an expert practitioner for your patients. Old-fashioned systems, process and procedures won't cut it any more. All nurses, including BME staff, have to become innovators, flowing with the tide, not against it.

'The perennial problem of scarce resources means that staff capable of devising new ways to provide cost effective services will be indispensable to their employers. You girls need to be looking for examples of how the best services are being delivered in other areas – or in other countries – and think of ways of introducing them where you are. If you can do that your jobs will be safe. We are in an age of research, technology and outcomes. If you can prove something works by demonstrating how you've achieved set outcomes, then you're home and dry. In fact you'll be headhunted. The secret of success,' she concluded as she poured herself another cup of tea, 'is always to be ahead of the game. Colour becomes irrelevant in those circumstances.' Judith concluded, 'this is the secret to keeping your job and progressing in it. Ascertain what needs to be done, forget the way you have always done it and make the changes. This will put you ahead of the game – and increase your market value exponentially.'

KEY POINTS

- ***Keep yourself up to date with information***
- ***Work smarter***
- ***Bring value to your work***

CHAPTER 5

Learn The Rules Of The New Game

Opportunity is missed by most people because it is dressed in overalls and looks like work.

Thomas Edison

DREAMS AND VISION

The three women warmed to their subject. There was reminiscence about the old times, conversation about the present and more than a little trepidation about the future. It was midday in no time, and Judith relocated the meeting to the kitchen while she prepared some lunch.

As they tucked into their tuna and sweetcorn sandwiches, they talked about the state of the NHS and the fact that many BME nurses still felt they had grounds to complain about discrimination. Judith assured them that there was a way forward - a method for career success that works for all, and which could be learnt. She related story after story of her time as a manager and how interaction with her peers had opened her eyes to how the higher echelons operate behind closed doors; how the game was played out, how cosy arrangements were made after work in restaurants and wine bars. She explained how people recruited within friendship groups. It gave them a sense of security, a feeling that their backs were protected.

'That's not fair' Jane exclaimed. 'So people miss out on promotion if they're not friends with someone at the top? Inequality is built into the system then, because there are so few BME at the top. They're usually the last to hear about any new initiative. Key information flow to them is either second hand or out of date, because they're not in the coffee room early enough in the morning for a tête à tête with the bosses. BME employees are habitually accused of rushing home and missing out on after work drinks and networking that goes on within teams.'

Judith picked up on this. 'If your home life doesn't permit elastic working hours,' she said, 'or you are not culturally comfortable with extracurricular networking, there are still ways you can be effective in the time that you spend at work. The directives coming from Government Central Office are emphasising the outcomes of your work. How effective is it? How beneficial is it to patients? You can raise your standing in the organisation if you become an outcome driven nurse. This is a major catalyst for success in any department. So, before you start a task, decide how you will measure your outcomes. "Vague" is not legal tender any more and anecdotal evidence is unacceptable. If you are being paid to deliver a service, ensure you provide one that is demonstrably cost effective, and you'll cease to be a casualty.'

Judith had it taped. 'The way I see it,' she argued, 'is that in the new economic and information age, nurses need to re-visit the dreams they started their career with. Recover that clear vision of what they want to do, how much they want to earn and where they want their career to end up. Then set the goals to achieve it. A plan will enable you to work your way from where you are now to where you want to be in the future. Jane, you're the youngest,' she went on. 'You need to be a visionary. Set time aside to think about your work and how you can improve the role you are in. Most people become stagnant, or they drift from one unsatisfactory post to another, allowing others to patronise them for a time. To be successful, you have to set opportunities to move into. Then, once you have decided what you want, propel yourself towards it, by working hard and being single-minded. You girls need to be aware of how fast things are changing in the profession and society as a whole.

'The Health Service operates differently from a few years ago. There is a constant search for better ways of providing care to patients. Don't think the bosses have all the answers. If you set time aside to learn, allow yourselves to be more creative and dream about your future I'm sure you could come up with ideas that will position you firmly in the inner circle.' With real enthusiasm, Judith set the scene.

'Can you imagine coming up with an idea that becomes the rallying cry of your unit, a means to raise team performance and achieve targets?' Sarah and Jane imagined what it would be like to have freedom to be creative at work: to introduce changes to make the ward welcoming to multi-cultural patients. The room was alive with possibilities. Sarah and Jane were projecting their own dreams onto the screen that Judith had erected. Judith smiled. She knew the impact she was having. 'One last piece of advice before I move on' she said, 'make sure you control the intellectual copyright of any great idea that you come up with. Each one of these ideas is another step on the ladder.'

PROBLEM-SOLVER

Although buzzing with the new horizons being paraded in front of her, Sarah returned to ground for a moment to remind Judith that nursing is still task-driven and can be hectic. 'Most wards run on adrenaline', she observed. 'The sheer workload means that it is very difficult to dream, or plan for change. We are immersed in our daily routines, going to work, working hard until we're ready to drop, and return home shattered. Then all we're fit for is dinner and bed. The next day we wake up and Groundhog Day starts again.'

Judith shook her head knowingly: 'Do you want to stop being a casualty? To break through the glass ceiling? If you do what you have always done, you'll get what you've always got. Change is a precondition of progress.'

After lunch, the three women returned to the front room and to look at the rather intimidating pile of documents on the table. Judith observed that rapid promotion was usually linked to problem-solving skills. 'The next time a problem arose at work', she advised, 'you women should have a go at finding a solution. Managers need solutions and if they come in people-shaped packages, then colour or creed is irrelevant.'

Judith gestured at the documents littered across the table. 'The mindset is to regard problems as opportunities,' she said encouragingly. 'When your colleagues moan about their work, just go and do it – and do it well. At times of pressure, volunteer to do extra. You'll soon be noticed and elevation will follow. Problem-solvers are the most valuable people in any organisation. The more problems you solve, the more adept you'll get at doing it, the better rewarded you'll be, and the faster you'll move on and up! Do this, and even if your career "Sponsor" leaves, you will have increased your employability. Be flexible about where you are prepared to work: The Health Service has numerous departments and the more experience you have the more employable you will become. Managers generally get to the top by knowing a little about a great deal of different disciplines. Don't be afraid to spend time outside the public sector. Nurses have excellent skills which are transferable and have a premium in other sectors'. Judith recounted how trouble shooters were recruited on high bounties to solve bottlenecks in the system.

'They came in, diagnosed the issue, prescribed a solution and sometimes implemented the cure. They are highly paid, spend relatively little time at the coalface and nearly always get home on time. Your analytical and problem solving skills will make you indispensable. If you don't already possess these skills, you girls need to develop them. They represent the secret ingredient of career success – and they separate victims from survivors. Which do you want to be?'

ADAPTABILITY AND FLEXIBILITY

Sarah and Jane had mentally answered that question. They were amazed at Judith's generosity, but the older woman seemed happy to be giving them all this priceless information and advice. She was like having their own personal 'deep throat' source about the NHS and what happened in it behind the scenes.

Judith continued, 'It's not always about what you know. In the main, it's about who you know and, most importantly, who knows you. If you're known, your name gets mentioned in the right places. If a manager is looking to fill a post, he or she will talk about it with other managers, and someone may know the "right" person for the job. In these circumstances the deal is done even before the job is advertised. The chosen one walks into a new job without lifting so much as an application form.' Jane was bursting to ask a question, her face colouring with indignation. Judith smiled and explained. 'Oh, the job is advertised and the recruitment process is followed, but the person discussed off record gets the job, no matter how strong the field.'

'And if you're not the chosen one?' Jane wanted to know. 'How do you break through the glass ceiling and get these opportunities?'

Judith responded, 'In the current climate, the competition is fierce. If you're not in the inner circle, you need to circumnavigate this by getting smart and working differently to the others. Curiosity, flexibility and a nose for which way the wind is blowing. These are useful skills. Do what you're asked, and then do more. As a director, I can remember asking people to do something and being told that it wasn't in their job description. That kind of rigidity spells death in an organisation like the NHS. What's needed is a "can do" attitude. Look carefully at your own working attitudes. If they have remained unchanged for years, or even months, start rearranging the fences. People who didn't bend when the wind blew used to be called rocks, nowadays they're more likely to be called barriers. Don't let them block your path'.

KEY POINTS

- ***Put your dreams into practice***
- ***Find solutions to problems at work***
- ***Be a team player***

CHAPTER 6

Design Your Programme For Success

To accomplish great things, we must dream as well as act.

Anatole France

SELF-LEADERSHIP

As Judith spoke, she could feel the nurses' frustration at the litany of injustices they had experienced. She could sense that they were feeling frustrated by their lack of power to make immediate changes and she wanted to send them home in a positive frame of mind. She passed a sheet of paper across the table and asked them to write down where they would like to be in five years professionally. The pair had no problem setting out their grand designs.

Judith read through them. 'Right,' she said, 'the work starts now. But before you implement your life plans, you need to be sure you're ready to make the necessary shifts in your own thinking. For the next part of the journey, you may want to move from a place where other people are blamed for any false starts in your career to a place where you are in charge. Ask yourself this question: Who is in charge of your life and the decisions made about it? Who is the boss here? Leadership starts by leading yourself through the change process. A leader may also want to manage their self-image, their self-esteem, and their self-discipline.

'Let's start with self-image. Why not have some honest conversations with yourselves? What might be the best way to build up your inner strength? If, of course, you want to stay focused and achieve your goals.

'And building inner strength can be influenced by weight. What would it be like to regain control of your shape? Have you decided what weight you want to be? Your general fitness is just one of the personal assets you may want to invest in if you are setting off on your path to achievement'.

Without getting drawn into the subject of weight control, Judith suggested monitoring eating habits, exercise, and sleep patterns. Judith knew that BME lifestyles with extended family and community commitments as well as work patterns can be significant factors in this area.

'Getting into shape,' she encouraged, 'makes you look and feel good and it increases your confidence. Another tip is to look the part you want to play. Research codes of conduct, including dress codes, of the people you aspire to emulate - then start behaving and dressing like them until it becomes a reality.

'Finally, get to know your strengths and weaknesses. Know what you are good at and what you like doing, and build on these. If you enjoy teaching, practice it. Ask to go on courses and get qualified. Then seek out opportunities to use these skills.

'Alongside building your strengths,' Judith continued, 'eliminate the false priorities, artificial imperatives and everything that shouts "important" when it isn't. Clear all the dead wood from your garden, winnow out anything that might suffocate your new goals.

Exercise your freedom of choice, choose the things you want to do wisely. Challenge yourself to do new things or to do familiar things differently, and then watch senior managers fight over your services.'

SELF DEVELOPMENT

The pitter-pattering sound was the scales falling from Sarah and Jane's eyes. They exhaled deeply, realising that they could achieve success in their careers in the NHS if they did things differently.

'Stop and reflect for a moment. Before you start attacking others for not helping you,' Judith pointed out, 'begin by helping yourselves. Invest in yourselves. Read, learn, train and become an expert. It's been said that hiding information from the black man is simple, put it in a book. Make yourselves the exceptions to that rule. You owe it to yourselves and your children. Read, read more and then read more besides. There is no short-cut to knowledge. The information you want exists in other people's heads and in the books that they have written so that we don't have to. So read, train and practise. There's no point jockeying for promotion if, when you're promoted, you fall off the saddle. That damages the chances of ten other BME who are swimming upstream in your wake.

'We've spoken about the speed of change. New technology based on new information that is immediately accessible once it has left the author's head. Your knowledge and skill base can be renewed and replenished constantly. They will be obsolete in two to three years unless you do so. However, greater demands mean greater opportunities. It means lifelong learning. Go deep into your chosen area. Read books, articles, magazines – become the source of others' enquiries.

'This equally applies to your job. Know what is going on around the world in your specialism and discover best practice that you can then replicate. Demonstrate this knowledge in your teams. Make yourselves indispensable at work,' Judith told them. 'This is how you grow tall enough to touch the glass ceiling, stop being a casualty and break through the glass.'

SELF-EMPOWERMENT

Judith observed a shift in attitude in Sarah and Jane. They were noting everything she was saying and were gratefully acting upon it. It was obvious that Judith was highly proficient in empowering people to excel professionally – and the fruits of her expertise were already evident.

The next vital ingredient, was focus.

'If you lose focus, you lose the battle. Be persistent and unswerving when you re-engage at work. It's going to be a bit of a shock to the system and will inevitably cause discomfort at times. You will be tempted to go back to the old ways or be deflected by outside distractions. Emulate those who you admire, but ensure that the drive to succeed comes from within. It will be hard work, but exhilarating. However negative the response, remain positive. It is your dream that you are building'.

Judith had been a manager in the health service. Part of her job had been to make changes in her relationships with work (including BME) colleagues. Judith had found some staff stepping up as allies in this process whilst others remained resolutely untractable in their ways. The secret was to find your own communication style and working modus operandi.

'Break your five-year plan into chunks. Then work on one segment at a time until you've arrived at your destination. Don't be deterred or distracted. Don't use colour as an excuse. Others won't make allowances if you allow your head to drop. Stay on course. Find ways to reorganise your workload so that you can get through more at less cost. Working out how to reduce waste and increase productivity, will bring you to the attention of those who can help you in your career. When you have reached this level you won't be ignored, far less discriminated against'.

KEY POINTS

- ***Lead yourself***
- ***Develop yourself***
- ***Motivate yourself***

CHAPTER 7

Break Through Time

Human beings, by changing the inner attitudes of their minds, can change the outer aspects of their lives.

William James

STOCK TAKING

Jane and Sarah sat in awed silence. Judith's words were nothing short of inspirational. What a day! Judith wasn't finished yet. 'Now,' she smiled, 'I'm aware of the time and we'll have to finish soon, but there is something important I need to tell you. I hope I've made it clear that you can take back control of your career path. Start by taking stock of your life now. Now move from that inventory to your future growth spreadsheet. Then identify the best route from your current position to your future one.'

Judith issued a second sheet of paper, and asked them to stocktake their lives, under the following headings: personal qualities, skills, interests, values, achievements and dreams. Judith advised the girls to be brutally honest with themselves in identifying what they had and what they lacked, so that they could begin to address the difference.

'It's important, no matter what stage you're at,' she explained, 'that you value yourselves, enjoy your lives, and consciously plan to achieve more. This exercise will highlight where the work needs to be done. It will flag up dormant resources that you possess. It will also illuminate unhelpful habits'.

Judith advised them that they could continue to work on their self-assessments when they got home. Most important was to record everything and commit to working through it. Then, once these qualities, skills and abilities were on paper, they could apply the necessary self-belief to make it happen.

'The history of BME staff in the NHS,' Judith said, 'shows that most of them have developed limiting beliefs. I've heard people explain that, because of their ethnicity, accent, name, age, education or colour they'll never be a director or a chief executive. But there are ways of changing these self-limiting beliefs to positive, unlimited ones.' She grinned. 'Ask me how another day!'

NEW STARTING POINT

'Based on our conversation,' Judith continued, 'it will be good to set down a new starting point for planning your career. Sarah, it's clear that you haven't been exposed to any strategic working. And Jane, you have just started working in the NHS, so we can short-circuit your progression into areas of your choice from this point on. There are lots of other pathways to follow, of course. Depending on your aspirations, you can follow the managerial route, the clinical leadership pathway, get involved in education, and these days, if you are business minded, you can form a social enterprise. These are just a few of the options available in the NHS, you can also tap into the private or voluntary sectors.

'Then, once you know what it is you want, you have to ask for it. Asking for what you want is one of the keys to success. Don't be passive. Ask. That's a sure way to get paid more. To prepare, start to seek opportunities in the organisation. Ask your line manager what you have to do to qualify for the next promotion or pay rise. Ask for the training you need, the exposure you require; ask to shadow someone doing the job you want; ask to be seconded to temporary roles, just for the experience. Ask for a sabbatical from your current role to try something new.

'Be persistent. Keep asking until someone listens. Ask politely but confidently, and wait for a response. If the answer you get is negative, ask what it takes to get a positive one. Take time to plan and execute your career progression. Let people know you're not going away and that you're happy to enjoy the same privileges as your non-BME colleagues.'

POSITIVE ATTITUDE

Judith looked at the clock. 'OK,' she announced, 'this is the last point I'm making today and then we can stop. You girls have got masses to do, and the next time I see you I want to hear about your progress.

'During my time in the NHS (and I doubt things have changed much), BME staff were labelled aggressive. The distinction between aggression and assertiveness is blurred in most people's minds. Knowing this, I would expect you two to differentiate between those two attitudes for the benefit of your peers. By all means argue your case, but do it with your head and not your heart. If you rely on emotion, you'll lose the argument. You will say things you regret. Your body language will let you down. Finger pointing and head shaking as a kind of semaphored disapproval will simply mean that managers won't want you in their teams. Be courteous - but firm. Be a person of your word. It matters.

'Be aware that your personal philosophy is impacted by the organisation you are in. That may be damaging to you, especially if it goes against your personal convictions. If this happens, decide whether you want to work within these paper walls, or whether it's time to rewrite the rules. This isn't always easy. Make sure that your career path matches your heart. Then your mind will follow.

'People are at the centre of everything we've talked about today. Everything we do is motivated by and for people. If you treat others as you would like to be treated, you will find success in everything you do. Someone once gave me an invaluable piece of advice: - they said, the more you are liked and respected, the more likely it is that doors will open for you.'

Judith sat back in her chair. She smiled at the reaction she had generated. You could almost hear minds whirring in the room. 'The next time you go to work, think about how you are going to improve the relationship you have with key decision-makers in your organisation.'

Sarah and Jane nodded in unison. This was good advice and something they could start doing immediately. Perhaps success in the NHS wasn't beyond reach after all. A new way of thinking and a smarter way of working could combine to make success possible after all.

KEY POINTS

- ***It's time to take control of your own destiny***
- ***Set goals to achieve your dreams***
- ***Your attitude will determine your altitude***

CHAPTER 8

Fast Track Your Success

Always bear in mind that
your own resolution to succeed is more
important than any one thing.

Abraham Lincoln

It was 5.00pm and Judith had been talking all day. Sarah and Jane were reeling with all the new information that they had been armed with. Judith motioned for them to sit back and listen for the last time. She wanted to summarise what she had been saying to them over the day.

'The message to BME staff in the NHS and other care professions is clear. No-one disputes that there is institutional racism running through society - including the NHS. Research by Government, the Royal College of Nursing and other bodies have confirmed this. It is undisputed that it is difficult for BME staff to progress into the boardroom, and they are over-represented in bullying, harassment cases and capability reviews, and are the most visible section of the workforce pursuing cases through employment tribunals'.

Yes, there are Government initiatives to address NHS failures on race and equality issues.

Targeted training and development opportunities via the NHS-sponsored 'Breaking Through' programme has undoubtedly had some impact in helping BME people reach senior positions in health and social care. In the case of nurses, the highly regarded Mary Seacole awards have assisted nurses to plough new ward care furrows for the specific benefit of BME patients.

This is vital progress, not only for the job satisfaction of BME employees, but for the wider public satisfaction in, and the reputation of, the NHS. New management teams that represent ethnic groups fairly are more likely to provide services suitable for minority patients and in so doing reduce inequality among BME staff, service users and carers.

At a crucial stage in this slow progress towards equality, the global economy took a downturn, pulling Britain into a deep financial crisis. The Government has responded by making ferocious cuts in public services. Job losses in our sector are inevitable and BME staff are likely to be more vulnerable than most, with a higher risk of losing their jobs or experiencing stasis than their non-BME counterparts.

Workplace protocols keep BME trapped under the glass ceiling. Job opportunities are denied to them, their talents are ignored, experience and expertise opportunities siphoned, information withheld, and their endeavours to progress thwarted. Staff who speak up during restructuring and mergers are often silenced, or worse, made surplus to requirements.

The career game has fundamentally changed in recent years, and BME need to adopt new rules if they're going to successfully engage in this game. This is new grounds. There is no need anymore to adopt the old guard's approach to life in the NHS. Rather than reactive, BME people can now be proactive and set their sights on the summit, rather than the foothills. More than this, you owe this activist mindset to yourselves, your peers and the community you serve. The imperative now is to develop skills that will enable you to enhance your role, and equip you to move into your next one.

Mastering the new game, developing a positive attitude and being alert to opportunity at all times is vital. There's no point adding to the problems of the organisation. Instead, be a problem-solver. Audit your attributes, set smart goals for your career, then focus on your plan to achieve these. Avoid seductive short cuts in training and education as there is no substitute for knowledge and experience.

Cultivate your visionary skills, anticipate events, and turn yourself into a leader – of yourself and others. Don't be afraid to ask for what you want and be prepared to take risks. Celebrate the success you gain along the way. Celebrate differences between people and use them to carve your own distinctive path towards a place when you can say you have fully explored your potential.

Be encouraged by the thought that where there is a problem, there is also an opportunity. BME staff in the 21st century, don't have to be casualties in the workplace any longer. You don't have to wait for somebody to give you the position you want. You can choose to climb to the top of the career ladder, and anyone who is ambitious has the right to be shown how to do that.

The route to a turbocharged working life includes adoption of the information super-highway. Those who don't embrace it will be left behind. The wise nurse who wants to move to the front of the pack should embrace change, and use it as fuel at work. Becoming a problem-solver with a reputation for retrieving poor performance in the organisation will propel you into the higher echelons.

Most importantly, invest in yourself. Be a lifelong learner. Read avariciously, train assiduously, and demand opportunities to progress you in your career. To fast track this process, look for a mentor or coach - someone who has done what you are aspiring to do. Be prepared to pay for assistance – it will be worth the price of admission. Although thin on the ground, there are excellent role models who BME staff can approach. These great BME achievers will, hopefully, be willing to support you and others that follow.

Express solidarity with your peers - don't tread on your colleagues to get to the top. Snitching, snivelling and being work averse will backfire in the long run. Work hard all the time, not just when the manager is watching. Form networks of support to share ideas and experience, and watch how that takes you forward at pace. Avoid a crab mentality - where we all scrabble to get out of the barrel but won't let anyone go first. As one of us begins to climb out, the others pull us down. For the BME to be taken seriously, we have to be seen to be speaking with one voice and supporting each other.

Treat people, all people, with respect. Be tolerant of others and embrace the diversity you see around you. Be true to yourself, be yourself more fully and never, ever try to become someone else. Cultivate skills that increase your likeability in the inner circle, yet enable you to remain yourself. Hone your communication, influencing and negotiation skills. These will deliver those promotions that you thought were beyond you.

Judith's big idea was networking. There is strength in numbers. Judith's advice for Jane especially was to join as many groups, forums and networks as possible. It works all the time in the 'old boys' networks. Groups enable you to share experiences, learn from others and connect with people who share interests with you. The girls were surprised that Judith advised them to join non-BME networks as well as BME ones. Judith pointed out that non-BME are experts at networking, team building and supporting one another. Job opportunities are the lingua franca and these conversations take place in networks. Become part of a broader network.

Ask for help. There is no shame in this. Curiosity leads to knowledge. Alliances lead to strength. There are frameworks in the NHS to assist you. Senior management is supportive when it makes good business sense for them and for you to progress in your career. The organisation will also benefit from your untapped talents and resources. Staff shortages and other exigencies may reduce your ability to network. But focus, energy and drive is self-driven so never use this as an excuse to give up.

Judith took a deep breath.

'All that's left for me to say is remember to have fun as you work hard in pursuit of your ultimate dream. Don't take life too seriously. We're playing games, not fighting wars. Some you win, some you lose, but don't give up. You play on until the final whistle blows and you have won.'

HOW FAR DO YOU WANT TO GO?

The aim of this book is to demonstrate that, with knowledge of the rules, you can progress from where you are to where you want to be, regardless of your colour or creed. My wish is for the insights in this book to awaken the creative and curious person in you, and accelerate your pursuit of your dream. The key is to take control of your own life and career. Don't wait patiently for an employer or a colleague to give you permission to progress. Track the opportunity, hunt it down and capture it. Be prepared to work tirelessly to achieve your objectives. If you put the suggestions in this book into practice, you will find your career inexorably moving into fast forward. The route to success is not as crowded as you may think. The limits you have placed on yourself may be someone else's construction.

Know your own mind. What is it that you want? Yes, that's right. That thought, there. Good. Now go and get it.

KEY POINTS

- ***Act now***
- ***Look for opportunities***
- ***Have fun on the way***

Publishing and Learning Resources

Shirley Baah-Mensah

CAREER ADVANCEMENT SPECIALIST

SPEAKER - TRAINER - COACH

If you've found this book helpful, why not recommend it to your friends?

Shirley provides training and consultancy to organisations to address equality and diversity issues within their workforce. We help employers comply with legislation and government policies on recruiting, retaining and developing staff from diverse ethnic backgrounds.

We also provide one-on-one coaching for staff who want to develop themselves and their careers to the full.

For further help or information, visit
www.nomorelimits.co.uk

Here you can also subscribe to Shirley's regular newsletters on personal and professional development.

To book Shirley for consultancy or as a speaker, contact 020 7078 7273

References

Access of BME staff to Senior positions in the NHS, NHS Institute for Innovation and Improvements, 2009 Issue: 185

http://www.library.nhs.uk/Ethnicity/ViewResource.aspx?resID=304598
Commissioning a Patient - Led NHS, Department of Health 2005.

Department of Health Equality Framework: Priorities for Action, 2003.

Equality and Diversity in the NHS - Demonstrating Best Practice for BME staff and Patients, Department of Health 2007

From Cradle to Grave: Fifty years of the NHS: Geoffery Rivett (King's Fund, 1997)

Improving working lives: black and minority ethnic staff networks: guidance, Department of Health 2001.

Many rivers to cross: The History of the Caribbean Contribution to the NHS Ann Kramer (TSO 2006)

Minority staff blocked from senior NHS roles. Health Service Journal, 2009

Minority staff get worse deal. Health Service Journal 2008

Releasing the potential within BME networks, Royal College of Nursing, 2006

Roots of the Future: Ethnic Diversity in the Making of Britain (Commission for Racial Equality, 1996)

The future nurse: the RCN vision, Royal College of Nursing, 2004